MW01267746

Cosmetic Counter Survival Guide

How to Buy the Right Skincare and Makeup

Third Edition
ISBN 0-9707290-0-6
Copyright © 2008, 2005, 2002 by Chris Scott
Makeup Gourmet®™
All Rights Reserved
printed in the United States of America

Book and cover design by Deborah Taylor
Author photo by Amy Scott

This book is dedicated to my parents Don and Sue
to whom I am eternally grateful and indebted to for all things.

Acknowledgements

It is an incredible joy to get this information out to the general public. In the process of making this book, several people helped to guide it towards completion. A very special thank you to my dear sister, Amy Scott, for lending her editorial advice and to Deborah Taylor, for her generous energy and inspiration in designing this book. Also, thanks to Mark D. Ryan for providing developmental support. All my love to Mary Jo for everything else.

Table of Contents

Table of Contents *(continued)*

Introduction: Is This Book For You?

Cosmetics can bring a lot of joy to life. Maybe you've experienced the pleasure of skincare and know how much soft and radiant skin can add to a healthy, confident appearance. Or maybe you've never experienced skincare but sense a desire to express more of yourself through your appearance. Either way, one thing is certain: the way we choose to look in the world is a very personalized, fun, and creative aspect of who we are.

Luckily for us, the world of modern cosmetics is super-abundant with high-quality products and variety and more people than ever enjoy the benefits of skincare. But for all its riches, the world of modern cosmetics has its drawback: too many people walk into the cosmetic section of a department store expecting to treat themselves to some well deserved self-care, yet leave feeling overwhelmed by choices, skeptical of product claims, and unhappy about their purchases. As someone who has worked in the cosmetic business for 20 years, I'm here to tell you, it doesn't have to be that way!

The purpose of this book is to demystify department store cosmetics to the cosmetic consumer. Upon finishing this book, you will be able to successfully navigate your way through any cosmetic department. Furthermore, you will have a working knowledge of which products are going to meet your needs.

There are common theories and strategies used by all cosmetic companies and once you become familiar with these similarities, you will see the cosmetic department in a new light. No longer will entering the cosmetic department be akin to embarking on a mysterious journey with unknown surprises around every corner. Instead you will gain a working knowledge of how the cosmetic industry operates, and this information will enable you to easily handle the overwhelming decisions that face you in the cosmetic department.

I am writing this book because after 20 years of serving the cosmetic needs of consumers, I realized I have a wealth of information. I am asked the same questions about makeup everyday. This book will give you as much knowledge, if not more, as the sales associates in the cosmetic department. I am not trying to minimize the cosmetic department employee. After all, they are the people with whom you will enter a relationship of trust when purchasing cosmetics, and they—and only they—can explain with specialized knowledge the uniqueness of the brand of cosmetics they represent. What I am trying to give you, the cosmetic consumer, is a head start so that you can talk with anyone in the cosmetic department while shopping for cosmetics and have some knowledge of the subject at hand.

Learning a skill is one thing, but mastering it takes lots of practice. Seek out those employees in the cosmetic department with lots of practice. They won't waste your time, and will be able to help you find the appropriate cosmetics.

I strongly believe in buying cosmetics at department stores for reasons I make abundantly clear in the following pages. I am not endorsed by any department store, nor do I endorse any particular cosmetic line, though as a consumer, I do have my favorites. In a few, rare instances in this book, I will suggest a particular cosmetic company. I only do this when a particularly hard-to-find product is made by only one company.

My goal is to illuminate the world of department store cosmetics for you so that you can find the products that fit your needs. Your own experiences in the cosmetic department will reveal to you which particular cosmetic brands are right for you. I say brands (plural) because I know no one who owns only one brand of cosmetics. Also keep in mind that every seven years our bodies recycle and have new sets of needs. If what you are using stops working, it is time to reassess your needs.

As to how to apply makeup, there are already many "How-To-Apply-Makeup" books out there. This is a "How-to-Select-the-Best-Skin-Care-and-Makeup" book, and I am confident that it will help you the next time you enter the cosmetic department.

Part One: Understanding Department Store Cosmetics

Department Stores, Beauty Supply Stores, and Drug Retailers

Is the department store the best place to buy cosmetics? Yes, yes, and yes. The advantages of shopping in a user-friendly department store far outweigh any trial and error you will experience at the drug or beauty supply store. Some of the advantages are:

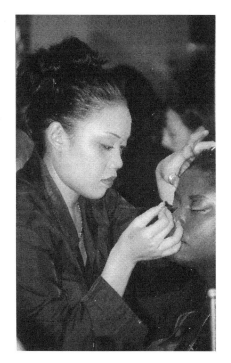

a). **Personalized attention.** Salespeople in a cosmetic department are trained to show you all the products they have in their line and how to use them. You are never wasting their time by asking questions and receiving makeup demonstrations. That is their job and, without you, they would be unemployed. It is acceptable and suggested to call the cosmetic counter(s) you wish to visit prior to your arrival. This way you can reserve an appointment especially for you and know that a counter person knowledgeable about the cosmetics you are interested in will be at your service upon your arrival.

Every line holds special events to promote their products. These services include facials, massages, seminars, guest makeup artists, video makeup application, etc. These services are almost always provided free of charge, or, the fee is redeemable in merchandise. Either way, the services provided are always complimentary. This is an excellent way to train yourself in makeup application. Check at different counters the next time you are in the cosmetic section and ask each line what its next event will be. You'll be amazed at the services constantly being offered, free of charge! This benefit alone more than compensates for the price difference between department and drug store cosmetics.

b). **Samples.** In this day and age, any cosmetic company that doesn't sample their product will not be around very long. Sampling gives you the opportunity to try everything before you buy. If samples aren't available, come prepared with small plastic containers to take home about a week's supply from a tester and try out the product for yourself. Always ask permission before getting a sample. Usually the line person will want to assist you in making your personalized sample (a line person is a sales person from the store who represents a particular line of cosmetics). Remember, it is to the line person's advantage to have you like their products.

c). **Return policy.** Cosmetic departments in department stores have a fairly liberal return policy. Find out what the policy is before you buy to protect your investment. Even with the best guidance and coaching, certain products will not work for you. It is better to be able to exchange or return an item than throw your money away by discarding your unusable product. This is another excellent reason to shop in a department store.

d). **Quality.** I will address the issue of quality versus price in the next section. Suffice it to say that the products you buy in a department store are of a higher quality than cosmetics available in drug stores and beauty supply stores. I am not attempting to say that drug store or beauty store cosmetics are worthless, because they are not, but I am making an argument as to why it is worth pursuing the best quality possible when it comes to products you put on your face.

The Dollars and "Sense" of Looking Your Best

There are people in the media who pose as the "consumer's advocate" and claim that the exact same ingredients are used to make the least and most expensive cosmetics. The theory is that all products produce relatively equal results. The argument of these "consumer advocates" is "Why pay more when the exact same combination of ingredients is available for less?"

It is important to differentiate between the quality of these ingredients. People who claim that there are no differences between one face cream and another are masquerading as the consumer's friend when they say "Buy the cheap stuff; it's the same as the expensive stuff." We all know this is just not so. Is there a difference between the quality of different makers of wines or chocolate? Of course there is a substantial difference. Both are made from

Remember: Department stores can afford to give you hand-and-foot service. Why not be pampered when you buy your cosmetics?

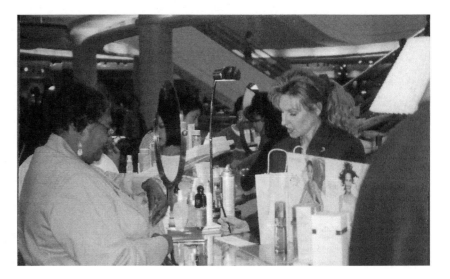

grapes or cocoa beans, yet some wines and chocolates are far superior to others in taste, texture and overall satisfaction.

Is every blouse the same quality? Forget about designer names for a minute; what are some of the differences between one blouse and another?

a). The type of material used

b). The type of pigment used to dye the material

c). The pattern of the blouse

d). The quality of thread, buttons, zippers, beads etc.

e). The feel of the blouse on your body

f). People's response to the blouse

What makes a quality product? It is the ingredients, the workmanship, and the expertise with which it is made. There is no mistaking a quality item. A quality product is made with precision, finished with refinement and endures. The distinction we need to make in our own budgets is what is affordable and unaffordable quality.

We all have different priorities as to what quality items we feel are most important. For some, it is a luxury car. For others, it is a preference of silk to rayon in their clothing. The majority of people I know hold personal appearance as a high priority. High quality cosmetics (meaning cosmetics found in department stores) can help maintain or increase our personal appearance. There are two advantages you have with cosmetic department cosmetics.

a) Though the cosmetic department face cream or foundation is more expensive than your drug store brand ($50 compared to $10), it is the absolute highest quality combination of ingredients that anyone's money can buy.

b) Most of us can afford that bottle of cosmetics far sooner than we can afford the luxury car of our choosing. We can have the best now.

When it comes to products I put on my skin, I care greatly about the quality of the ingredients that I apply to my face. Cosmetics are an area where we can afford the best quality money has to offer.

Does that mean that the most expensive product is always the best for you? First, let it be known that the cost mark-up for cosmetics from the manufacturer through to the consumer can be as high as 500%. Once that is accepted, there is a difference in quality compared to price up to a point. Let me share a quick story:

Remember: Most of us can afford that bottle of cosmetics far sooner than we can afford the luxury car of our choosing. We can have the best now.

Once in Manhattan I slipped into the Versace boutique. A jacket caught my eye and the salesperson helped me try it on. To this day, I have never looked as good, nor has any piece of clothing looked as good on me. The price was twice what I ever dreamed it would be. I have never looked as good in a piece of clothing since. Did I buy it? No. My entire assets didn't add up to the price of that coat. I have since worn jackets that looked good and were affordable, and I buy them. Yet in my heart I know that nothing wears like designer goods.

I firmly believe that designer products are higher quality products. Will another brand do? Of course it will. It is up to your own prioritization to decide for yourself in what things you want the best. For some it is cars; for others, it is clothes or wine or perfume or whatever. And there are those who only want the best cosmetics. Dollar for dollar, the designer makeup isn't 100% better than other makeup. Half the extra amount you pay for designer cosmetics is for the quality, and the other half is the name. You cannot get one without the other.

The products that are the most important in terms of quality are: (1) skincare, (2) foundation and (3) powder. Everything else is a matter of taste.

Probably the best and most used argument in the cosmetic department about whether you should buy an expensive cream for your face is "You only have one face." Though this may sound like the ultimate fear tactic to sell cosmetics, it is true. Our face is the first thing people see when they look at us. The appearance of our skin and the appearance of the cosmetics we choose to wear say a lot about who we are. The rest of our bodies are usually protected and disguised by clothing, but our face is all alone up there on top of our bodies. It is important to treat that exposed part of our anatomy to the best that we can afford.

Within the cosmetic department there is a wide price range available. You don't have to buy the *most* expensive product to receive high quality. There are eye liners that sell for more than $25 and those that sell for less than $5 within the cosmetic department. In later chapters I will detail what the generally accepted priority products are. Suffice it to say that the appearance of the skin is the most important function of your cosmetics. This is achieved by using the best skincare, foundation and powder you can find.

It is impossible for me to make a generic statement as to which product or brand is the best for you. The advantage is yours when shopping at the department store. All products are available for sampling and complimentary demonstration. Ultimately, you need to judge which cosmetics feel and work the best for you. I have clients whose skin is radiant and glowing when they use Clinique (a relatively inexpensive line). I have other clients who can only use the higher priced products (such as La Prairie or Sisley). Both clients attain equal results yet they pay a dramatically wide price difference for their products. It is not so much the price of the product but your individual needs that determine the correct product choice for you.

Yes, cosmetic department cosmetics are more expensive, but remember, you really do only have one face. Service, quality, return policy and samples come with every product you purchase. Cosmetics are an affordable luxury, you put them all over your face, and you should prioritize highly which cosmetics you wish to wear. You would not throw your designer silk dress in the washing machine to save a few bucks. You know that would ruin it. Why are some people willing to take that chance on their face?

The quality of ingredients you receive in department store cosmetics can make the difference in the life of the appearance of your face. Your face is not a place to compromise. Budget your money to include quality products for your skin, the same way you'd budget money for medical care, dental treatments, and eye exams! It is worth it.

Mastering the Maze of Different Cosmetic Lines

Why are there so many cosmetic lines? Money! Cosmetics is a multi-billion dollar industry. To gain even one percent of this industry's gross profit is to be extremely financially successful. Lauder, Inc., figured this one out long ago and has created or acquired niche lines to fulfill the unique requirements of the customer's varied needs. Under the Lauder, Inc., umbrella alone is Estee Lauder, Aramis, Clinique, Prescriptives, Lab Series, Origins, M.A.C., Bobbi Brown, La Mer, Aveda, Jo Malone, Bumble and Bumble, Darphin, American Beauty, Flirt!, Good Skin and Grassroots. By diversifying, Lauder, Inc., is the cosmetic heavyweight at the moment.

Cosmetics are disposable products that need constant replenishing. It is worth the risk of the cosmetic entrepreneur to create a makeup line, then hope that you buy from it. Don't be discouraged by the quantity of choices. Instead, take comfort in the options available and follow my step-by-step process to find the best products for you.

In order to find the cosmetic line that suits your needs, ask yourself, "What is my 'look'?" Every cosmetic line has a "look," or an image. Some are strong and unmistakable. Others are more subtle and less defined. Your initial reaction to how a line presents itself should inform you if these products are the right ones for your "look."

So what is your look? Are you "natural," "professional," or "glamourous"? Chances are you are probably each of these looks at one time or another. It will

Remember: If you were given only one garment to wear for your entire life, how would you treat it? Consider your face that one garment. You only have one face. You may be able to alter it surgically, but you can never exchange it. Treat it at least one hundred times better than your finest piece of clothing.

save you time and money to know what you want from your cosmetics before you buy them. Evaluate your needs, then buy the cosmetics that will fulfill those needs. It is as simple as that.

In order to fulfill your needs, you may find that one line alone does not satisfy your multi-faceted makeup wardrobe. This is a time to rejoice at the options available to you! If your varying needs are subtle, however, you will probably find almost everything you need within your line of preference.

Discontinued and Limited Edition Items

There is nothing more frustrating in cosmetics than expecting to pick up your tried-and-true lipstick only to find out it has been discontinued and is no longer available. The relationship some people have with their favorite makeup is parallel to their hair stylist. You've searched long and hard to get the results you want and then someone takes it away from you. Don't take it personally; it is the nature of the cosmetic business. Let me explain first the philosophy behind discontinued items and then next the economics.

Philosophically, makeup, like shoes and clothes and handbags and accessories and so on, is part of fashion. Though we may not follow all the new trends, it is an accepted phenomenon in the fashion world that styles change and that it is very exciting to watch it change. Many people would not dare wear last year's style when this year's so strongly clashes with its predecessor. Why then is makeup expected to stand still while the rest of the fashion world moves on? It can't. That is not its function. Makeup is designed to accentuate the person and the fashion of the moment. Artistically and stylistically speaking, if you keep wearing the same look, be it in clothes or makeup, your look eventually will become dated. Because makeup companies sometimes set the trend for color, it is vital that cosmetic lines constantly reinvent themselves to find new ways to combine and formulate the new colors of each season.

Sometimes, in this process of reinvention, older colors are discontinued to make room for the new ones. Cosmetic companies can't hold on to every style of makeup, the same way the clothing department doesn't keep displaying summer styles in winter. It doesn't mean the colors that are discontinued are invalid; rather, the cosmetic companies need to make room for the new. Generally, the overall sales performance of a product is the main factor on whether it is discontinued or not. This is the second part of the equation: the economics. Never take it personally that your color was discontinued—it has nothing to do with

Remember: In today's world, we are often asked to be many people. The variety of cosmetic lines can help fulfill that need.

your taste. Cosmetic companies look at their overall high sellers and keep them in their collection. Those that fall below a certain percentile are economically expendable and discontinued.

So how do you protect yourself from this phenomenon? I have a couple of tips. When you know you love a color and will wear it forever, ask your salesperson if that color is soon to be discontinued. If they don't know, find out where that company is headquartered and call them up. If it is about to become discontinued, buy as many as you can and store them. Dry cosmetics (e.g., eye shadow, blush, powder, etc.) seems to last forever. Just put it in a cool dry place sealed in an airtight plastic bag and your product will be their waiting for you when you want it. If the product is wet (e.g., lipstick, foundation, moisturizer,etc.) still seal the products in an airtight plastic bag and store in refrigeration. Don't freeze it, but keep it refrigerated. These items won't last forever, but a good long time. Remember that makeup is like food, when it spoils, it gives off a foul odor. If your makeup smells sour or like rotten eggs, toss it.

Your other option when a color is discontinued is to be bold and go find a new one. There are so many options in the cosmetic department, there is bound to be at least five other colors similar to yours. Stay open minded. This is a good time to maybe even find a better color than your discontinued one. I know that you may prefer one line over another and that may limit your options. Still, within your cosmetic lines of choice, there are still a lot of options when looking to replace a color.

It is also important to note that seasonally some colors are released as limited editions. Limited edition means that the cosmetic company has manufactured a set number of a particular item designed to sell out during that particular season. Limited editions are definitely trendy colors that go with the theme of that season. Often the most unique ideas and formulations are offered in a limited edition and it seems crazy that, economically speaking, the cosmetic company wouldn't make more, but they don't. If a particular limited edition is extremely successful, chances are you will see it in a more standardized form in later seasons. Also, some companies will copycat a great idea. One company will do an outrageously successful limited edition and another company will pounce upon the idea and issue their own version of it ASAP. That means if you really want that limited edition product and missed out the first time around, keep an eye out, another company may come out with it sooner than you think.

To avoid any rude surprises, always ask when buying a product you like if it is a limited edition or a discontinued item. This is a surefire way to avoid the disappointment and inconvenience of finding out your favorite lipstick is no longer made when you attempt to replenish.

Remember: Always ask when buying a product you wish to continue to buy if it is a limited edition or a discontinued item.

Remember: Competition breeds higher quality products and better service.
It is to your benefit that there are many cosmetic lines available to the public.
Each new line puts the pressure on the existing lines to improve.

Gimmicks to Avoid

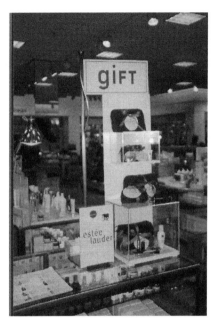

Ask cosmetic companies if they are glad they ever started gift-with-purchase offers and they will all answer with an emphatic "NO!" The gift with purchase, or as they say in the business, GWP, was a sales promotion that was more successful than anyone's wildest dream. It has gotten to the point that many consumers will not buy cosmetics unless there is a gift attached. There are also consumers who buy cosmetics not because they need it, but only because they are getting something for free along with their purchase. Because of this, the perceived value of cosmetics has decreased because the product you are purchasing no longer stands on its own.

When cosmetic lines are offering gifts, their sales are extraordinary. Once the sale is over, they fight to maintain customer loyalty. Cosmetic companies wish they could stop offering any GWP. The problem is that they have created consumer expectations, and are not willing to take the financial hit to stop offering the GWP. The truth is that the GWP promotions are so expensive to offer that the companies make very little profit. Even if their customer is loyal only when they offer a GWP twice a year, they are not willing to give up that sale. Thus, the cosmetic companies have created a vicious cycle that they must continue, though in their hearts they would love to never offer another GWP.

Why am I telling you all this? Because I want you to buy the best cosmetics for you, not for a free gift. If it turns out that the product that works best for you is also offering a free gift, then count your blessings. Otherwise, don't compromise your face for a gift that usually contains only a few, if any, products you truly desire anyway. Stay clear-minded and buy what you want and need, not what is being given away. It is better to stay focused and leave the cosmetic department with only the products that are best for you.

Cosmetic Counters vs. Open Sell

Traditionally, when shopping for cosmetics in department stores, you approached a counter, peered through the glass case that held the products, and waited to be waited upon. If you have shopped for a lipstick in the last five years, you have probably encountered a "new" type of retail layout in the cosmetic department at certain stores. Someone finally got the bright idea (maybe after shopping at the drugstore) to put all the cosmetic products in reach of the customer. The idea is simple. Let people select what they want without having to wait for the attention of a salesperson and get on their way.

I have experienced all types of reactions to the old (counter) vs. new (open sell) way to cosmetic shop. Some find the new method (open sell) a bit more chaotic and disconcerting while others love their new-found freedom. I have clients who wax nostalgically about how they use to shop at the counter. There are others who have taken to the open-sell concept praisingly and have never looked back. From a salesperson's point of view, the new open-sell concept is a bit more challenging. Customers can now approach their "counter" from many directions and it is often impossible to know who was next. It is important as a customer and to your benefit to know the kind of attention you want before you go shopping, then choose the type of selling environment that best fits your needs.

Here are three basic profiles of shopping preferences and the different selling environments which best serve these profiles.

Remember: If it is attention you want, call ahead and make an appointment. If it is only product replenishment you need without waiting your turn, an open- sell environment is best for you.

1. **Counter service only:**

   · You like to be waited upon.

   · You trust the opinion of your salesperson emphatically.

   · You don't mind waiting your turn, and in return you get the full attention of the salesperson when it is your turn.

   · You may enjoy services like complimentary makeup applications.

   · You may like to be called on the phone from your salesperson.

   · You likc to look more than touch.

2. **Open-sell department store:**

   · You like to be waited upon or not.

   · You trust the opinion of your sales person to a point.

   · You want to get what you need and get out without having to wait for who-ever was there before you.

   · You may enjoy services like complimentary makeup applications.

   · You may like to be called on the phone from your salesperson.

   · You like to touch as much as look.

3. **Open-sell cosmetic-only stores**

   · You don't need or especially like to be waited upon.

   · You have your own opinion about what cosmetics are right for you.

- You want to get what you need and get out without having to wait for whoever was there before you.

- Services like complimentary makeup applications are not a priority.

- You probably don't like to be called on the phone from your salesperson.

- You like to touch more than look.

Depending on what your needs are, different stores may meet them more completely. If you need to pick up a quick mascara, run into an open-sell store, get what you want, and leave. If you are looking for more personalized attention, call ahead to the open-sell department store or counter service department store and make an appointment with your favorite person before you go shopping.

Part Two: The Basics of Skincare

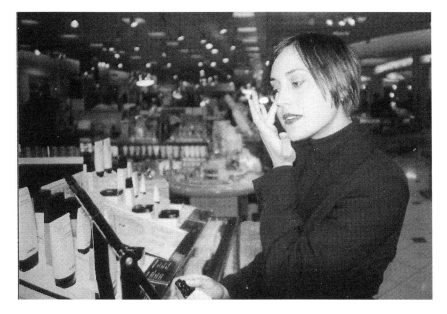

Remember: Variety is the spice of cosmetics. All cosmetic companies want to make their product more effective than their competitor. Shop around. The best products for your skin's particular needs are out there.

Sorting Out All the Products

Why are there so many skincare products? Skincare is big business, and new skin needs are always being discovered. The cosmetic companies pounce upon any new discovery to create a product to fulfill that need. All skincare products are a reaction to what the consumers say they need. Cosmetic companies know this simple marketing rule very well: "Fit the product to the market, not the market to the product."

It is far more expensive and risky to convince consumers that they have a certain need, and should therefore buy their product. It is far easier, safer, and more profitable to listen to what consumers say they need, then give the best argument why their product is the perfect solution.

For example, the term "anti-aging" would not exist if no one asked for it. Most everyone wants to look younger, and reversing the effects of aging is one way to achieve that. Yes, cosmetic companies have an overwhelming amount of products to fulfill your every skincare need, but they are only responding to what is being asked for by the entire consumer base and supplying it in the most convincing form possible.

Be patient and take time to sift through the different products each line offers. Trust your own intelligence. Read the box. It will state in a straightforward fashion what the key features and benefits are for each product. In later chapters I will explain what the basic skincare format is and how all these extra "special interest products" can fit in to your regular regime.

How To Read and Evaluate Your Skin

You know your skin better than anyone else. In most cases, you know the history of your family's skin. Look at the skin of your parents and grandparents. This is your gene stock. Whatever skin your parents and grandparents have or had, you have. Some people will appear as if their skin has never aged and they may have used only olive oil on their face. Others may appear 10 or 20 years older than they are despite the fact that they do everything they can to protect their skin from the appearance of age. Most of us fall somewhere in the middle. Everyone's skin is different, yet there are enough general similarities to create an effective skincare system that works for almost everyone.

Here are some basic questions to ask yourself. Based on your answers, you will have a working knowledge of your skin type. Knowing this will assist you when you approach a cosmetic counter looking for any skincare products.

Your skin is at its most balanced state when you first wake up after a full night's sleep. Remember that high amounts of alcohol or salt consumption can greatly alter the appearance of your skin in the morning. Hot weather conditions can produce a more oily skin type and cold weather can produce a drier or dehydrated skin type. Keep these factors in mind as you evaluate your skin. How does your skin usually appear in the morning is the question you need to ask yourself. It is best to write down your answers to the following questions so you have a list of information from which to work when shopping for cosmetics.

1. What is the feel of your skin to you in the morning? Does it feel comfortable, oily, taut or tight?

   If your skin feels comfortable, the balanced state of your skin is normal. Normal skin means you have an equal and adequate amount of water and oil on the surface of your skin.

   If your skin feels oily, the balanced state of your skin is oily. Oily skin means you have more oil than water on the surface of your skin.

   If your skin feels taut or tight, the balanced state of your skin is dry. Dry skin means that your skin has a low level of water and oil on the surface of the skin.

   If your skin feels oily across the forehead, down the nose and on the chin only, you have a *combination* skin. This is also called T-zone skin because the oil appears in a T shape on the face. Combination skin can have normal or dry cheeks to accompany the oily T-zone. If your cheeks are normal, it is best to treat your skin with oily skincare products. If your cheeks are dry, it is best to mix your products using oily skincare products on the T-zone and dry skincare products on the cheek area.

2. The only other factor you need to be aware of is whether your skin is sensitive or not. If your skin tends to react within the hour to certain products, you have sensitive skin. A reaction can be a burning sensation that doesn't go away, redness or bumps, and sensitivity to extreme hot or cold weather conditions. It is important to include in your skin type whether you are sensitive or not. Once again, only you know whether your skin is sensitive or not, and it is your responsibility to tell the cosmetics salesperson helping you exactly what your skin type is.

Once you know your skin type, you can approach any cosmetic line and ask what products they have for your particular needs. With this knowledge, the line person will focus only on products that fit your skin type, and you won't feel overwhelmed with a counter full of bottles staring you in the face.

Please circle your skincare profile below.

My skin type is:

NORMAL   OILY   DRY

T-ZONE W/NORMAL CHEEKS   T-ZONE W/DRY CHEEKS

I   **am**   **am not**   sensitive

Demystifying Skincare

Almost all skincare lines follow the same formula:

1. Cleanser

2. Toner

3. Moisturizer

This is the European skincare law in cosmetics. There are a couple of lines that work slightly outside this theory (Erno Laszlo, Janet Sartin). Regardless of this, as long as you know your "skin type" you are way ahead of the game.

Let's break this down to better understand the purpose of each step.

1. **Cleanser.** The purpose of a cleanser is to remove any dirt, oil, makeup or anything else that has accumulated on your face during the day or night . You want a cleanser that cleanses efficiently according to your skin type. You also want a cleanser that is more gentle than a body cleanser because you want to pamper your facial skin. Pampering is what will help your skin look its best.

The type of cleanser you choose often comes down to your personal preference. There are cleansing bars, cleansing gels, cleansing milks, cleansing oils, etc., available. Drier skins tend to prefer a milkier cleanser and oilier skins prefer a more thorough gel or bar. Regardless, use what feels good to you and is suggested for your skin type.

Remember: You only have one face. Treat it at least one hundred times better than your finest piece of clothing.

2. **Toner.** This is probably the most mysterious skincare product to the consumer. I hear almost every day "What does a toner do?" "Do I really need one?" The truth is you don't need any cosmetic product, but the reality is we look better if we use them. That said, toner is one of those products that the consumer didn't ask the cosmetic companies to make. It is a time-tested European skincare step that makes all of your skincare work better. Toner is usually a combination of water, witch hazel, vegetable extracts, sometimes alcohol for oily skin and other soothing and calming ingredients (specific ingredients depend on the maker). Toner provides the following two benefits.

   a. It follows up the cleansing process and picks up any trace debris the cleanser missed. (You may use a more gentle, less moisture-stripping cleanser if you know you are following up with a toner.) It assists in the cleansing process, thereby making the cleansing process more gentle. If your skin type is normal to dry (or sensitive), you want a non-alcohol toner. It will follow up the cleansing process without stripping the skin of its moisture. If your skin tends to be oily (and is not sensitive), use a toner with alcohol. The alcohol will kill bacteria that breeds in oily pores and creates skin problems. All people with sensitive skin should use non-alcohol toners only.

   b. Your toner makes all other skincare products you put on your face work better. It primes the skin to receive and absorb your moisturizer. The better you prepare your skin, the more receptive it will be to the products you apply. This means you receive the best results possible from all your other skincare products when you use toner.

3. **Moisturizer.** Beauty is only skin deep. Well, so is your skin. Simply put, the layer of skin that cosmetic products touch is only the very outer layer. The outer layer of skin has already lived in the deeper layers and is now dying. The function of moisturizer is to make this dying skin die a slow, graceful, beautiful death. The average life cycle of a skin cell is 21 - 35 days; after that it's all new skin. Dying skin cannot maintain moisture well, and unfortunately, skin cells without moisture make your skin look dull, weathered, and aged. Adding moisturizer to this top layer of dying skin plumps up the dying cells and makes them look their best before they fall off your face.

This description may seem rather graphic, but it is necessary to know if you want to understand the purpose of cosmetics and how to use them effectively. Cosmetics help us look our best, temporarily. The fact that our skin is constantly replacing itself makes it necessary to continually use skincare to make our skin look its best, and thereby use cosmetics effectively.

The world of cosmetics has its own vocabulary that you need to be familiar with in order to get what you ask for. The following is a table of skincare terms and benefits.

Skincare Terms	Benefit
Cleanser—cleans the skin.	Removes surface grime that can accelerate the effects of aging.
Toner—follows up cleansing and prepares skin to receive moisturizer better.	Skin is cleaner and more receptive to products.
Moisturizer—adds water and oil to the skin as needed according to your skin type.	Surface skin cells appear more radiant and skin looks and feels smoother. Skin also wears makeup better.
Serums- Special interest product that provides a concentrated dose of active ingredients to target micro-specific skincare needs.	Areas of concern are more acutely addressed providing improvement where you want it most.
Eye cream—moisturizes the eye area. Eye cream should be considered a maintenance must. This area has no conventional oil glands and is one of the first places we can see the appearance of age on our facial skin. Eye area tissue is very thin (only two layers where most of our skin has three layers) and requires a highly refined product that can penetrate a very thin tissue. Only eye cream can do this. I strongly encourage you not to put anything next to your eye that isn't ophthalmologically tested. By law, all eye creams must be ophthalmologically tested or they cannot be called eye creams.	The eye area appears softer, gains more surface elasticity and wears makeup better.
Exfoliate—removes surface dead skin cells (hopefully dead, although some scrubs are too aggressive and remove living cells as well).	Exposes living skin cells that by nature have a smoother, more luminous appearance, thus creating a more youthful appearance to the skin.
Alpha hydroxy/glycolic acid—a derivative from either lactic, citric or fructose acid that loosens dead skin cells. This makes the removal of dead skin cells an easier and more constant process. This ingredient also lightens the appearance of age spots and pregnancy masks. (Pregnancy masks are areas of darker pigmentation on the face caused by pregnancy.)	Produces a smoother, younger, clearer appearance to the skin.

COSMETIC COUNTER SURVIVAL GUIDE   PART TWO: THE BASICS OF SKINCARE 17

Skincare Terms	Benefit
Sun protection factor–protects the skin from photo-aging. About 80% of premature skin damage is from the sun. This product also protects skin from sun spots and possible skin cancer.	Produces a smoother, younger, clearer appearance to the skin, and reduces the risk of skin cancer. (This ingredient can protect your skin from accumulative damage as well.)
Anti-oxidants–neutralize the effects of pollution and free radicals on the skin.	Produces a smoother, younger, clearer appearance to the skin. (This ingredient can protect your skin from accumulative damage as well.)
Cleansing mask–usually a kaolin clay mask that absorbs excess oil and residue in pores and minimizes pore size.	Prevents break out, removes blackheads, and makes skin appear smoother and brighter.
Moisture masks–adds intense hydration to the skin in a short amount of time.	Creates the appearance of a smoother, luminous, softer skin (especially helpful to people who live in cold weather, are frequent flyers, or lead stressful lifestyles).
Exfoliation (enzyme) mask–a gentle mask that dissolves dead skin cells from the face without physical aggression.	Creates a smoother, softer, more luminous skin. This product is excellent before makeup and self-tanning products.
Mud masks–mud is full of minerals that create a healthier environment for the surface skin cells.	Produces a softer, healthier looking skin.
Retinol–an over-the-counter form of retin-A (vitamin A).	Produces a rosy glow and a more youthful appearance. Reduces large wrinkles, brown spots and surface roughness such as acne scarring.
Salicylic Acid–an over-the-counter treatment for acne.	Effectively decreases inflammation and the formation of new whiteheads and blackheads.

Skincare Quick Look Guide

SKIN TYPES	CLEANSER	TONER	MOISTURIZER (A.M. and P.M.)	SPECIAL CARE
NORMAL	Milk Bar Gel Oil	No Alcohol	Lotion Eye Cream	Cleansing Mask Moisture Mask Exfoliation
DRY	Milk Gentle Bar Gel Oil	No Alcohol	Cream Eye Cream	Cleansing Mask Moisture Mask Exfoliation
OILY T-ZONE & NORMAL CHEEKS	Bar Gel Oil	Alcohol	Oil Free Lotion Eye Cream	Cleansing Mask Moisture Mask Exfoliation
OILY T-ZONE & DRY CHEEKS	Gentle Bar Gel Oil	Alcohol T-zone	Oil Free Lotion T-zone Lotion Cheeks Eye Cream	Cleansing Mask Moisture Mask Exfoliation
SENSITIVE/ NORMAL TO DRY	Milk Gentle Bar	No Alcohol	Gentle Lotion Eye Cream	Cleansing Mask Moisture Mask
SENSITIVE/ OILY	Milk Gentle Bar	No Alcohol	Gentle Oil Free Lotion Eye Cream	Cleansing Mask Moisture Mask Exfoliation

Cosmetics and Dermatology Side by Side

Remember: Cosmetics and dermatology work hand-in-hand. Each does what the other is not designed to do and are therefore perfect complements.

Quite often I am approached by customers with medical questions about their skin. These questions can include inquiries as to why their skin has little white bumps; how to get rid of broken capillaries; what acid peel is right for them; should they use retin-A? It is important to understand the difference between cosmetics and dermatology.

Cosmetics are designed to help the surface appearance of healthy skin look better and, in some cases, provide prevention from accumulative skin problems (as is the case with sun protection and anti-oxidants). Skincare falls in the category of preventive maintenance, like flossing and exercise. There is nothing medical about cosmetics. Do not waste your time, try to save money or risk your health trying to solve serious skin problems in the cosmetic department. That is not the purpose of cosmetics. Beyond that, your cosmetic line person is not a dermatologist. In an attempt to be helpful, the line person may offer advice that may be considerably ill advised.

Dermatology, on the other hand, treats those conditions that require correction. Remember the old saying, "An ounce of prevention is worth a pound of cure"? We would all rather prevent problems from arising. Sometimes, regardless of how much you brush or floss your teeth, you get a cavity. The same can be said for skincare. Sometimes, the needs of your skin supersede the capacity of the cosmetic department.

Many dermatologist think that cosmetics are a joke because they pretend to offer the answer for troubled skin. Cosmetic companies know their place and never suggest that their products are more effective than what a dermatologist might prescribe. Instead, cosmetics can be used to prevent the problem from happening so you won't have to see a dermatologist.

Dermatologist approach a skin problem as a particular need to be solved. They disregard the rest of your skin to treat the problem for which you are seeking relief. This is to your benefit. If you have acne scars, you would love to see those scars disappear. The dermatologist will give you something to reduce the physical appearance of acne scars. The drug may work great; however, the side effects may wreak havoc on the rest of your face (in this case, usually intense dryness) Don't blame dermatologist for drying out your skin; they are only attempting to correct the problem that you have presented to them. In a couple of months, once your acne scars begin to disappear, you will feel much better about the appearance of your skin.

It is not the dermatologist's job to give you perfect, cosmetically refined skin, but rather to correct the problems that may arise with your skin. A nice benefit of cosmetics is that they can supplement your dermatologically prescribed regime. Cosmetics can help minimize the negative symptoms experienced when following a dermatologist advice to correct a skin problem. For instance, if a drug is drying out your skin, you can get high quality moisture enhancers to reduce the appearance of dryness on the skin. Or if you are having facial peels to reduce the appearance of lines and the skin is reddened, foundation can reduce the appearance of the redness until the discoloration subsides. It is always a good idea to check with your dermatologist about whatever supplementary products you decide to use on your skin. As long as what you use in addition to your dermatological regime does not create negative side effects, and it makes you feel better, use it.

So my answer to cosmetics versus dermatology is that cosmetics and dermatology work hand in hand. Each does what the other is not designed to do and are therefore perfect complements. Be thankful that both exist and be clear what your needs are before approaching one or the other. It will save grief, time and money. Better yet, you will get the results you seek.

Personalized Skincare Strategies

We all wish we could improve at least one aspect of the appearance of our facial skin. Common complaints are lines and wrinkles, age spots and pregnancy masks, blotchiness, dullness, oiliness, dryness, breakout, loss of elasticity, darkness and puffiness around the eyes, etc. With so much on the wish list, cosmetic companies have made problem-specific products (or special interest products) to address individual needs and wants. If you have a particular need above cleansing, toning and moisturizing, tell your line person and he or she will show you what is available.

Here is a trick. If you don't want to run from counter to counter comparing one product to another, find a neutral person (meaning someone without line loyalty such as a cosmetics manager, a beauty director for the department, a well informed friend, or a beauty magazine) and seek an opinion. They may lead you to what you are looking for quicker.

Special need products can be very effective and can greatly accelerate the improvement you are looking for in your skin. Most often these special interest products are called serums and they are more highly concentrated doses of the active ingredients that are designed to deliver improvement of your specific concerns. There are many to choose from so be picky-be specific-try before you buy- and expect results. Don't forget, you can sample anything.

The following is a list of common special interest skincare needs, along with types of ingredients and/or features that will offer the desired results. When you are looking to solve a special interest skincare need, check to see if the product contains the correct ingredients or claims the features mentioned below.

Lines and wrinkles, loss of elasticity—products that can remedy these problems include alpha hydroxy acids, retinol, anti-oxidants, intense moisturization, high sun protection factor, firming masks and temporary line softeners.

Age spots, pregnancy masks, blotchiness, dull appearance—products that can remedy these problems include high sun protection factor, alpha hydroxy acids, retinol, skin whiteners and exfoliators.

Oiliness, breakout—products that can remedy these problems include oil-free bases, oil controlling ingredients, salicylic acid and kaolin clay masks.

Dryness—products that can remedy these problems include high moisturization, hydration boosters, moisture masks, and high sun protection factor.

Note: Hydrating your skin usually means adding water to it. Even the oiliest skin can be dehydrated and crave water. Hydration products are for everyone. Moisturizer usually involves an oil-in-water molecule that adds oils as well as water to the skin. Normal skin has an even ratio of oil to water in the skin.

Darkness and puffiness around the eyes—products that can remedy these problems can include botanical extracts that encourage circulation by stimulating the outer layer of skin. Increased circulation of water and/or blood reduces puffiness and darkness, respectively.

It is in your best interest to find products that have blended your specific needs in as few products as possible. For instance, if you need high moisturization, sun protection, alpha hydroxy acids and line softening, try to find a product that contains all of those features. Your skin is very thin and can only absorb so much. The more complex your products, the more effective your skincare products will be.

Daytime Treatment vs. Nighttime Treatment

Your skin has different needs during the day and during the night. Salespeople are not trying to double their commission when presenting you with nighttime products as well as daytime products. The distinct differences between daytime and nighttime skincare are:

Daytime—a lightweight moisture formula is designed to sit lightly on the skin, acting as a cushion and a slide-prevention to your makeup. Daytime skincare carries environmental protection such as sun protection and anti-oxidants to guard your skin during the day. The goal of daytime skincare is to protect and prevent damage to your skin while helping to maintain your makeup.

Nighttime—enriched nighttime formulas are designed to produce greater benefits to the skin while you are at rest. Sleep is a recovery period for the entire body, including the skin. The products you use at night are designed to enhance the positive effects of a night's sleep on the skin. Because you are not worried about makeup sliding off your face or being shiny while you sleep, you can wear products that offer your skin much better results. Usually these products are more emollient and may have a shiny or opaque appearance. Blood flows closer to the surface of the skin while you sleep. Though the products bought cosmetically don't reach the depth of blood flow, they can enhance circulation in the skin, promoting a general state of healthy well being in your skin.

Generally speaking, if you want to buy only one product for each purpose of the skin, buy daytime products because they can also be used at night. Prevention, which is found in daytime products, is critical to the health of your skin. When you want the optimal benefits of skincare, invest in night-time products. Ideally, own both daytime and nighttime products

First Proper Products, Then Proper Usage

Now that you know which products work for your particular skincare needs, how and when do you use them? Your line person probably informed you in detail when and how to use each product. Even though everything made perfect sense in the cosmetic department, sometimes it all looks the same when we get home. The following chart shows a basic skincare regime that should work well with your products.

Most products are concentrated and do not require a large amount to be effective. Moderation is the principle when caring for your skin. Skincare is like exercise—a little bit every day will maintain your health. By the way, cardiovascular exercise and diet are other positive ways to nourish your skin, but that's another book.

DAY	NIGHT
1. Cleanser	1. Cleanser
2. Toner	2. Mask—if mask is to precede toner (see the instructions that come with your product)
3. Special interest product, usually called a serum, that is designed to precede moisturizer (see the instructions that come with your product)	3. Toner
	4. Mask—if mask is to follow toner (see the instructions that come with your product)
4. Moisturizer	5. Special interest product, usually called a serum, that is designed to precede moisturizer (see the instructions that come with your product)
5. Eye cream	
6. Special interest product that is designed to follow moisturizer (see the instructions that come with your product)	6. Moisturizer
	7. Eye cream
7. Makeup	8. Special interest product that is designed to follow moisturizer (see the instructions that come with your product)
	9. Sleep

Part Three: Makeup 101

Thinking it Over: Your Own Makeup Interview

And now for makeup. The following questions will help you decide which makeup items you actually want and/or need in your cosmetic wardrobe. In the same way you defined your skin type, there are a few basic questions you need to ask yourself to define your makeup needs.

Please ask yourself these questions. It is best if you write down your answers so you can use this worksheet when you choose your products.

1. When do I wear makeup? When do I want to wear makeup?

2. What is my skin tone, hair color and style, and eye color?

3. What are the makeup colors I love on me?

4. What are the colors I dislike on me?

5. What are the colors in my wardrobe (break this down into seasons of the year if your wardrobe rotates)?

6. What is my style of dress (casual, professional, night club, night at the opera)?

7. What is the range of makeup looks I require? The three basic looks are soft and natural, professional and finished, and glamourous and dramatic. Of course there are gradations between these looks, but these are good ranges to work with.

8. Do I need one, two, or all three of these looks in my cosmetic wardrobe?

9. How much time am I willing and able to give to the application of each look?

By now you should have a clearer idea of your personal makeup needs. Now let me help you find what you need in the cosmetic department.

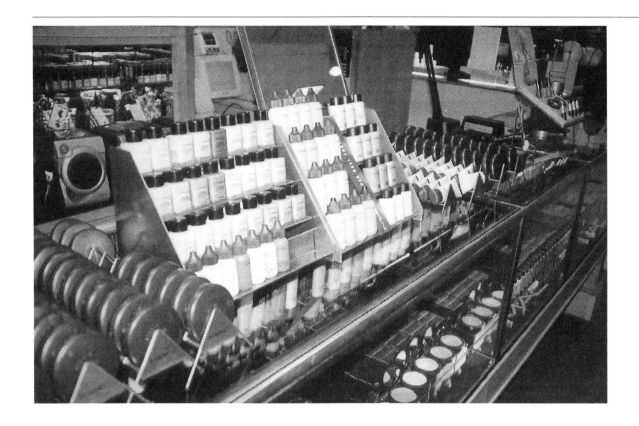

The Source of Lasting Elegance: Foundation and Powder

Great makeup can be compared to making a beautiful cake. If your cake is already good, the icing just adds an overall smoothing and uniformed appearance, and the cake decorations just add style, point of focus and color. Likewise, if your skincare is already good, makeup just smooths your appearance and adds fun, attractive touches.

After completing your skincare, the first item of makeup you need to consider is foundation. The purpose of foundation is to smooth the appearance of the skin and offer a more even skin tone. In reality, the best foundation look neutralizes the skin tone so that the colors chosen for lips, eyes and cheeks don't compete with any skin discoloration.

Everyone has different coverage needs and wants. The types of foundation and powder *coverage* (meaning degree of neutralization) available are:

· Sheer coverage
· Medium coverage
· Total coverage

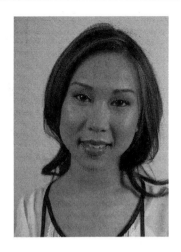

The types of foundation and powder *finishes* (overall look of the skin) available are:

· Matte (no shine) finish
· Semi-matte (subtle glow) finish
· Dewy (all-over glow) finish

For a *soft and natural* look, it is best to use sheer coverage with a dewy or semi-matte finish.

For a *professional and finished* look, it is best to use medium or total coverage with a semi-matte finish.

For a *glamourous and dramatic* look, it is best to use total coverage with matte, semi-matte or dewy finish.

Let's first talk about the types of foundations available that offer these different types of coverage. Keep in mind that the technology for cosmetics is very advanced; consequently, most formulas are water based even though they contain oils. If people say their foundation is water based, it does not necessarily mean it is oil free: it means that water is the highest proportioned ingredient in the foundation.

Oil-free	This is usually the sheerest form of foundation available. For a dewy finish, do not powder this foundation. For a semi-matte finish, powder with a translucent (non-opaque) powder.
Liquid	Liquid usually means it is a water-based foundation that also contains oil. Oil provides better bonding to the pigment in the foundation, thus better coverage. This formula provides medium coverage and should always be set with a powder to control the oil in the foundation. A translucent powder will provide a semi-matte finish and an oil controlling powder will create a more matte finish.
Cream	Cream is the richest of foundations. It is ideal for dry skin types who want a more hydrated look to their skin, or for someone who wants total coverage. A translucent powder will provide a dewy to semi-matte finish and an oil controlling powder will create a semi-matte to matte finish.
Pancake	This looks like a dry, very dense powder. It is water activated and applied with a sponge. It is a very popular form of theatre Makeup but is also used widely for everyday Makeup. It can be set with translucent powder. The coverage is total, and the look is very matte.
Powder	Do not confuse this for pancake or translucent powder. Powder foundation is opaque (solid color), provides coverage, and varies in its finish. Some powder foundations can only be applied dry (without water). Others have higher coverage if applied with a damp sponge (like pancake). Since this is a powder already, it does not require a powder finish. This foundation can provide a sheer, medium or total coverage and usually has a semi matte to matte finish.
Stick	A cream stick of foundation that provides all levels of coverage. It is an easily portable form of foundation that provides higher coverage than its powder counterparts.

Normal Skin—any one of these foundations will work for you, depending on your needs.

Dry Skin—you usually want to get a more luminous look to your skin. Liquid or cream makeup will work best for you. If you are allergic to any type of oil, keep in mind that you can still use oil-free makeup and use hydration enhancers on your skin before you apply your foundation.

Oily Skin—you usually want to control the shine with a more matte finish. Oil-free,* liquid, pancake or powder are the best foundations for you. Keep in mind that some cream-like foundations are highly refined and may smooth your skin better than some matte foundations. You need to powder with a more oil controlling powder to maintain a matte look if this is the case.

Unless you are allergic to oils, I believe that oil-free liquid foundations are not the best choice for severely (oily 24 hours a day) oily skin. Because there is no oil in the foundation, when the skin produces its own oil, it more easily separates the foundation on the surface of the skin. Remember, water and oil do not mix. Foundations with a small amount of oil absorb your own natural oil better and do not separate so quickly in the presence of new oil produced by your skin. Oil-free powder foundations are appropriate and effective for all oily skin types.

Matching foundation to skin tone is vital. Once you find the formula you want, try three tones of the same foundation that most closely match your skin tone. Apply them vertically on your jaw line, smoothing them down under your jaw line and into your neck. Blend them as much as you would

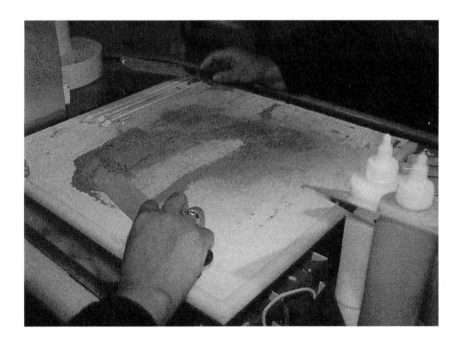

anywhere else on your face, then wait a minute. Waiting gives the foundation time to set up and react with your body's chemistry. Find a good light: halogen is best, fluorescent is worst, and, if you can, step outside into daylight with a mirror and see which foundation shade blends the best from your jaw line into your neck. Whichever shade blends the best is the one you want to choose.

Some people want a lighter look to their skin. It is okay to pick a lighter foundation. Some people want a darker look to their skin. It is not okay to pick a darker foundation. Instead, use a bronzing powder to add the color you desire over your matching foundation. Cosmetically speaking, it is flattering to have foundation lighter than or matching your neck color, but when foundation is darker than your neck color, your foundation is no longer inconspicuous.

Once you have selected your foundation or foundations, you can move on to powder. I mentioned powders with foundations because they determine the foundation's type of finish. The purpose of powder is to set (dry) the foundation while smoothing the foundation more closely to the skin. Except for the few exceptions already mentioned, consider powder, even if only a small amount, a requirement. Powder not only dries the foundation, it enhances the productivity, longevity, and effectiveness of the foundation. Without it, foundation falls apart in an hour. With it, foundation lasts all day.

Translucent powder is the best and most common form of powder used to set foundation. It is ideal because, although it does create a more refined look to the foundation, it doesn't mask the appearance of the skin created by the foundation. Many of my clients cannot stand a powdery look, which is why translucent powder is so ideal. It sets the foundation without imposing a heavy or powdery look to the skin.

Powder comes in different forms for different reasons:

Loose	This form is best to use and keep at home and is usually a better monetary value. Loose powder is easier to manipulate whether you want to use a puff or a brush to apply.
Compact	The sole purpose of compact powder is convenience. After all, one thing loose powder does not do well is travel. Loose powder is so fine, even the best travel container has trouble controlling it in transit. A compact powder is usually slim, has a mirror, and is convenient when you want to refresh the finish of your foundation or control excess shine. Most companies sell whatever loose powder you use in both a loose and compact form. They are not two different powders: the compact has just been highly pressed so that it does not fall apart when in transit.
Matte	Some powders contain a high percentage of talc or other oil absorbing ingredients to give and maintain a more matte finish. This is ideal for people who want to control oily skin and/or maintain a matte finish.
Light	There are powders that contain highly refined reflective ingredients that create a more luminous, even glow-like effect on the skin. This powder is ideal for those people who want to brighten up a dry skin or maintain a luminous finish.
Bronzing	This usually comes in compact form. Brush this over your set foundation or alone to give a more suntanned look to your skin. This is also the most natural way to make your skin tone appear darker. Even a small amount of this powder can give you a "healthier" appearance.
Correction	These are distinctly tinted powders to balance out the color ratio in your skin: **Green** neutralizes redness and/or blotchiness in the skin. **Rose** or mauve brightens up an otherwise sallow skin. **Yellow** warms up golden tones without changing the skin tone the way a bronzing powder does.

Powder also comes in different shades, though not nearly as many shades as foundations. If your skin is light, get a light powder. If your skin has some color though is by no means dark, get a medium powder. If your skin is dark (not including skin of people of color) get a deep or dark powder.

People of color need to find a line that caters to their skin tone. Unfortunately, the cosmetic industry does not cater to people of color nearly as well as those with western European skin tones. Although I do not endorse any one cosmetic line, the MAC, Fashion Fair, Bobbi Brown, and Prescriptives cosmetic lines have an excellent range of powders for people of color.

Foundation & Powder Quick Look Guide

Foundation Formula	Coverage	Finish
Oil-Free	Sheer	Semi-matte, Matte
Liquid	Medium	Dewey to Semi-matte
Cream	Total	Dewey to Semi-matte
Pancake	Total	Matte
Powder	Sheer, Medium, Total	Semi-matte, Matte
Stick	Sheer, Medium, Total	Semi-matte, Matte
Powder Formula	**Coverage**	**Finish**
Loose	Sheer, Medium Total	Semi-matte, Matte
Compact	Sheer, Medium, Total	Semi-matte, Matte
Matte	Medium, Total	Matte
Light Reflecting	Sheer, Medium	Semi-matte, Matte
Bronzing	Sheer, Medium	Dewey, Semi-matte
Correction	Sheer, Medium	Semi-matte, Matte

Creating Your Bouquet of Color

The dilemma of finding the best makeup colors (eyes, lips, cheeks) for you can be a difficult experience. The following discussion about what color is and how it works will hopefully free you when selecting colors for yourself. My hope is that you will discover the range of colors that is both appropriate for you and not at all restrictive.

There are three major headings to consider before knowing what are appropriate colors for you.

a. Your natural color intensity

b. Soft and Natural, Professional and Finished, Dramatic and Glamourous makeup

c. Your wardrobe color intensity and range

To decide what makeup colors to wear, coordinate them with your wardrobe, hair, skin and eye color intensity. When I refer to intensity, I mean the lightness or darkness of a color: low intensity is a very light color and high intensity is a very dark color, and medium intensity is somewhere in between. It is just as important to know what intensity of color (low, medium or high) is appropriate for you as the type of color (meaning orange, blue, etc.). Color is generally dictated by fashion (what you wear). Intensity of color is dictated by your natural color intensity.

Your Natural Color Intensity

It is best to understand the natural color intensity of your face without makeup before making makeup color choices to enhance it. There are three factors to consider: hair, skin, and eye color intensity. In each of these categories your natural color intensity is either low, medium or high. Once you are familiar with your natural color intensities, you will know what intensity of makeup color you need to create a desired effect.

First let's consider hair. If you are a person who is blond, light gray, white haired or any other natural or dyed color with similar depth, your hair color intensity is low. If you are a black, dark brown or any other natural or dyed color with similar depth person, your hair color intensity is high. All other colors between these two extremes are considered medium.

This same formula applies to eyes and skin. If your eyes or skin are light, they are low intensity. If your eyes and skin are dark, they are high intensity. Anything between these two extremes is considered medium intensity. When I speak of eye color, I am referring to the center of the eyeball that surrounds the pupil. Remember, when considering eye color intensity you must look at the depth of value of your eye color. If your eyes are a pale blue or light green, they are low intensity. If your eyes are a deeper blue or green, they are a medium intensity. Any type of eye color can have more than one intensity. Do not assume that all blue eyes are low intensity and all brown eyes are high intensity. What shade of blue or brown are they? Try to judge the intensity of the color rather than the color itself.

What are your color intensities? Please fill in the blanks. Your answer to each blank is either low, medium or high intensity.

_____ hair color intensity

_____ skin color intensity

_____ eye color intensity

Soft & Natural, Professional and Finished, Dramatic and Glamourous Makeup

The intensity of color you choose to wear will dictate the natural, professional or glamourous effect you are attempting to create. When designing a look for yourself, remember:

· For a *soft and natural look*, choose an intensity of colors that is equal to your natural color intensity;

· For a *professional and finished look*, choose an intensity that is one level higher than your natural color intensity; and

· For a *dramatic and glamourous look*, choose an intensity that is as far from your natural color intensity as possible.

Remember: Low intensity is a very light color and high intensity is a very dark color, and medium intensity is somewhere in between. Try to judge the intensity of the color rather than the color itself.

Note: To achieve a dramatic look, you don't have to wear the darkest makeup imaginable. High contrast is dramatic. If you have a low-intensity skin tone, wear high-intensity color. If you have a high-intensity skin tone, wear low-intensity color. If you are a medium-intensity skin tone, go as far as you can in either the high- or low-intensity direction.

Now that you understand your natural intensity of colors, it is easier to select intensities of color to achieve your desired results. The closer a color intensity is to your natural intensity, the more natural it will look. The farther away a color intensity is to your natural color intensity, the more dramatic the result.

For example, if your skin, hair and eye tone are all medium intensity, then medium-intensity lipsticks and eye colors will appear natural on you. If your eye color intensity is low and you apply the same medium-intensity eye makeup to your eyes, your eyes will appear more dramatic because the intensity of the color of the makeup is in contrast to your eye intensity. If your eye intensity is high, the same medium-intensity eye colors will not provide substantial contrast to your natural eye color and appear less effective.

High-intensity contrast is another thing to consider. If you have a low intensity skin yet have high-intensity hair (like Uma Thurman in *Pulp Fiction*), it is possible to wear a medium- to high-intensity lip color and still look natural because of the negligible contrast between hair and lip color. Also consider a high-intensity skin with platinum blonde (low-intensity) hair. Even though a high-intensity lip color can create a natural effect if the hair is also high intensity, with low-intensity hair, the high-intensity lipstick will appear much more dramatic.

Still there is the question as to which color to choose. Sure you may know the right intensity of color, but should you choose pink or orange? How do you decide? Luckily you have a big clue in your wardrobe closet.

Your Wardrobe Color Intensity and Range

The other part of the equation to factor in is your wardrobe. Since what you wear usually covers 80% of your body, it is important to incorporate your wardrobe color choices with your makeup color choices. You may wear different wardrobe pieces throughout the changing seasons depending on where you live. Also keep in mind the texture of the fabric you prefer. Are you a more quilted person? Do you prefer more flat or light reflecting material? The matte or reflective quality of your wardrobe should be reflected in your makeup.

What is the difference between a warm and cool color? The difference is that some colors have more of a yellow base whereas others have more of a blue base. Yellow is a warm color, like the sun. Blue is a cool color, like water. There is also another family of colors called neutrals, which have a balance of yellow and blue in the base, and are appropriate with any wardrobe. In order to create a balanced color story between your face and body, it is important to try to work within one of these color "families" for each look.

Wardrobe and makeup color choices can be put into four categories:

1. **Neutrals**—white, beige, tan, brown, camel, ash, bone, taupe, gray, charcoal, black, etc.

2. **Warm Sun**—yellow, gold, lamé, maize, orange, copper, bronze, peach, terracotta, etc.

3. **Cool Violets**—royal or navy blue, purple, violet, magenta, burgundy, teal, rose, plum, etc.

4. **Rose-Blue**—pink, coral, salmon, watermelon, rose, etc. (these colors are a combination of Warm Sun and Cool Violets in varying degrees).

Also, any combination of the above colors encompasses the endless possibilities that are wardrobe color choices. For the most part, we know what wardrobe colors we like on ourselves and what wardrobe colors we don't. There is no formula as to why you like yourself, say, in green and not purple. It is just your personal preference. For some reason you feel and look better in certain colors more than others. Based on the wardrobe color choices you have made, it is important to supplement your wardrobe with complementary makeup colors and intensities. Remember, your wardrobe falls under the same low-, medium-, and high-intensity rules as your natural color intensity.

Here is where the intensity equation becomes more dynamic. Let me play out a few scenarios so you can play the intensity game along with me.

Low-intensity facial features: Let's first start by considering a person with low-intensity hair, eyes and skin. For a natural look, she should wear low-intensity colors. If her wardrobe for spring was predominately pink and blue, she needs to wear low-intensity colors from the Rose-Blue family. What if she prefers to wear royal blue and deep fuchsia in her wardrobe? In order to maintain a natural look that does not wash her out, she will need to pick more medium-intensity makeup colors from the Rose-Blue family to complement the intensity of her wardrobe. If she wants to look dramatic for evening, she then goes into high-intensity makeup colors in the Rose-Blue family. If for some reason she likes a particular orange sun dress, she needs to choose the appropriate intensity makeup colors from the warm color family.

Medium-intensity facial features: Now let's consider a person with medium-intensity skin and eyes with high-intensity hair. She only wears light neutrals in her wardrobe. Because there is already a built-in contrast between her wardrobe and natural color intensity, she needs very little color to finish her look. Colors that match her natural color intensity will look appropriate and fresh. For more drama she can raise her makeup color intensity a little. If she decides to wear black, then she needs to raise all of her makeup colors to a higher intensity to keep her colors balanced.

High—intensity facial features: Last let's look at a person with high-intensity skin and eyes with medium-intensity hair. She loves to wear bright purple and violets. In order to balance her skin intensity with her wardrobe intensity, brighter medium-intensity makeup colors from the Cool Violets family will complement her look best. To appear more dramatic, lower-intensity eye color (for example, pearly white or rose) will brighten her eyes. Also, a high-intensity eyeliner will add lots of dramatic detail to the look.

These are just some hypothetical examples of how different combinations of intensities dictate the types and intensities of colors to choose when coordinating makeup with wardrobe.

Contrast in intensities can regulate the effect of the makeup colors you choose. For example, peach and soft brown have similar intensities, and when they are worn together, they achieve a soft look because the intensities between the two colors vary little. Black and white, on the other hand, have high opposing intensities, and when they are worn together, the contrast creates a dramatic look because the intensities vary widely.

Today's hair styles sometimes will bring a dominant color into the picture like bright red or purple burgundy. When considering color for yourself, also examine if you have a more extreme hair color. If you do, by all means find makeup colors that work together with your hair color. In my experience, regardless of the wardrobe color choice, if the hair color is extremely dominant in a conventional or non-conventional way, it is best to use the hair color as a guide to your makeup color choice and not your wardrobe.

I have helped more than 100,000 people select the right combination of colors and intensities. No one is exactly the same. Everyone has different needs. It is important to constantly ask yourself the same questions when shopping for makeup.

· What is my natural color intensity for skin, hair and eyes?

· What is the color and intensity of my wardrobe?

· Do I want a natural, finished or dramatic look?

Anyone can wear any color. The question is which intensity of these colors best suits your natural coloring and wardrobe. Within each color family, there is an infinite range of intensities. One of these intensities will be right for you, depending on your natural coloring and wardrobe.

You want to balance the intensity between makeup and wardrobe. If you are wearing a pale blue wardrobe, a light pink or rose will probably balance well as a lip color. However if you are wearing navy blue in your wardrobe, a deeper plum or blue red will appear more appropriate. As long as you work within the same color family and parallel intensities of color, your makeup color choices will be correct.

It is always more cosmetically correct to under-dress your makeup than over-dress it. If you are torn between two colors, fearing one may be too strong for your taste even though it matches the intensity of your wardrobe, it is better to go with the lighter shade. Coco Chanel said "Less is more," and it couldn't be more true when choosing makeup color intensities for yourself.

Natural Color Intensity Quick Look Guide

	Low Intensity	Medium Intensity	High Intensity
SKIN TONE			
Natural Look	L	L/M	M/H
Finished Look	M	M/H	M/H
Dramatic Look	H	H	L/H
HAIR COLOR			
Natural Look	L	L/M	M
Finished Look	M	M/H	M/H
Dramatic Look	H	H	H
EYE COLOR			
Natural Look	L	L/M	M
Finished Look	M	M/H	M/H
Dramatic Look	H	H	L/H

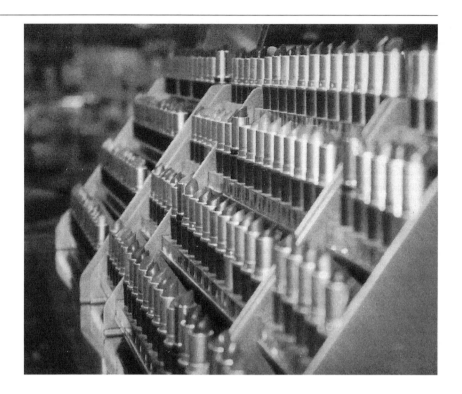

Let Your Lips Lead The Way

Now that you have selected the foundation and powder you need, let's move on to lipstick. I like to pick lip color first when doing makeup because it sets the tone for the rest of the look and provides a basis from which to balance all other color choices. In my experience, if a woman does not like her lipstick, she does not like her makeup. It is imperative to find a color that you like and that complements and enhances your facial features and wardrobe. Please review the color chapter earlier if you need to refresh your understanding about how to select colors.

There are many formulas of lipstick available, each boasting its unique features and benefits. The following chart summarizes the types of lipsticks available and what to expect from their performance.

Gloss	Gloss is usually a sheer or slightly tinted gel that gives a wet look to the mouth. Gloss can be worn alone for a more natural look or over lipstick to heighten the lipstick color. Gloss can make the lips appear softer, especially if your lips are prone to dryness or aging. A high-power shiny gloss can be very dramatic. In most cases, a gloss look is very sexy. Gloss is available in wands, pots, and stick form. Be aware though that gloss will wear off your lips fairly quickly.
Sheer	Sheer lipsticks have more color than glosses and usually have a semi-gloss finish. Sheer color is not opaque so it mingles with your natural lip color to create a soft lipstick look. Sheer lipstick is designed for a natural look and for weekend makeup. Sheer lipstick usually comes in stick form and, although it is longer lasting than gloss, it too has a short lip life.
Cream	A majority of all lipsticks sold are cream lipsticks. Cream lipsticks have a higher concentration of pigments and create an opaque color on the lip. The creamy texture softens the look of the lips, but the glow from the formula is minimal. Properly applied, cream lipstick wears very well.
Matte	Matte means no shine at all. The concentration of pigments are usually highest in this form of lipstick and it is usually the longest lasting lipstick you can wear. Because of matte's severe anti-shine design, lips can appear dry and cracked and some mattes dry out the lips even further. It is important to hydrate your lips well if you are a matte lipstick wearer. The matte look is definitely dramatic on the lips and can create a highly refined, almost untouchable appearance to your makeup. There are some matte formulas that are not so severe in their dryness. It is best to test a few to see which formula suits you if you wish to wear matte lipstick. Matte lipstick is available in stick, cake (applied with a wet brush), pen (goes on wet, dries to a matte) and pencil.

Frost	Frost is an additive that can be blended into any of the previous formulas to add a reflective shimmer to the lips. Some frosts are highly refined and add a subtle shimmer. Other frosts are more glitter-like and have a mirror-ball effect on the lips. Lip color can be pre-frosted, but frost is also available on its own to add to any lipstick. Frost comes in gloss or powder form.
Pencil	Some lip colors come in pencil forms. The penciled look tends to be more matte and is longer lasting, which is good for people who want long lasting color. Some pencils are also waterproof.
Lip Liner	Besides using lip pencils for lipstick, there is a product, usually in pencil form, known as lip liner. The purpose of lip liner is to define the shape of the lips, minimize or enlarge their appearance, correct the appearance of off-sidedness, and enhance the intensity and longevity of lipstick. Lip liner creates a highly effective look to the lips and the lipstick, and if you are going to use it, choose a color that is of equal or higher intensity than the lipstick, and choose a color that is in the same color family as the lipstick. Lip liner can also change the appearance of the color of the lipstick with great results. For example, using a red liner with a coral lipstick, when well blended, provides a high-intensity lip color. There are infinite possibilities between lipstick and lip liner. Be creative, remember what color base you are working with, and have fun. Neutral lip liners such as brown or taupe naturally intensify the shape of the mouth and work with almost any lip color. Neutral lip liners tend to soften the intensity of the lipstick on the lip, whereas non-neutral liners tend to intensify the lipstick color.

If you are looking for a lipstick and are not sure what your wardrobe will be, it is best to go with a neutral color. Also, if you want your lipstick to brighten up your eye color, keep this in mind:

- Blue eyes are enhanced by rose, pink or bronze tones.

- Hazel and/or green eyes are enhanced by violet/plum tones.

- Brown eyes are enhanced by coral, peach, burgundy and purple tones.

Speaking of eyes, once you have selected your lip colors, it is time to find appropriate eye color to match.

Lipstick Quick Look Guide

Lipstick Formula	Finish	Longetivity
Gloss	Sheer & Shiny	2 - 4 Hours
Sheer	Sheer & Moist	2 - 4 Hours
Cream	Opaque & Hydrated	4 - 6 Hours
Matte	Opaque & Dry	4 - 8 Hours
Frost	Pearlescent	2 - 6 Hours
Pencil	Opaque & Dry	4 - 8 Hours
Lip Liner	Opaque & Dry	4 - 8 Hours

The Infinite Expression of Your Eyes

I will present the products available to you for the eyes in the order I feel they should be applied. Please keep in mind that eye makeup is where you can be your most expressive, and for every suggestion I make, there are an infinite number of variations on that suggestion. Therefore, I will try to stay mainstream with my suggestions and digress only when it is absolutely necessary.

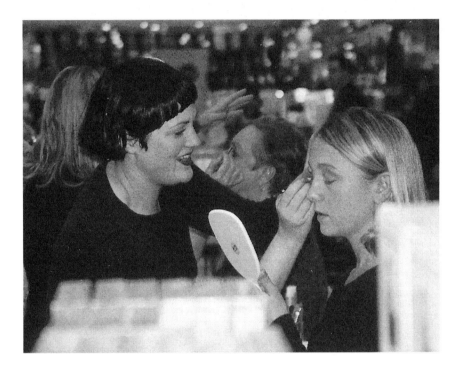

Eyebrow	The first area of attention should be your eyebrow. A groomed and shaped eyebrow almost immediately brings a near-finished look to the eye. Pencils and powders are the most common makeup tools used to enhance your brow. Be sure to have a brow brush to blend and better manipulate your eyebrow product. Find a color that matches your hair color. You can go a little lighter, but for most purposes, do not go darker than your hair color on your brow. The only exception is for a blonde. Because it appears naturally in nature, blondes can go as dark as they want on their brow and it is never a makeup faux-pas. Also available are brow gels, which come clear or tinted. These gels hold the shape of the brow and can give them a conditioned look. Most brow gels come in a mascara-type dispenser format and are quick and convenient.
Eye Shadow Base	This products neutralizes the skin tone around the eye area and provides an ideal environment for eye shadow to blend well and last without creasing or melting. Eye shadow base usually comes in a cream-to-powder or plain powder format. Find a base that matches or is slightly lighter than your skin tone. Most companies that offer eye shadow base have at least three shades to choose from. Even if you do not intend to wear eye shadow, eye shadow base does wonders for creating a clear appearance to the eye area and whitening the whites of the eyes.
Eye Shadow	Eye shadow colors are sold in singles, doubles, trios, quads, quintets and so on. The word to remember here is shadow. You want to create the illusion that your eyes are superbly lit by creating just the right shadow to enhance your particular eye shape. All shadows found in nature have two parts: light and dark. Your goal is to find the best light and dark shadows for you, considering which look you want (natural, finished, or dramatic) and what color family you are working within (blue-base, yellow-base or neutral). Any additional shadow colors beyond light and dark can serve as a gradation between the light and dark shadows for a better blended look.

Eye shadow comes in the following forms. When it comes to eye shadow remember: *blend, blend, blend!*

Cream	Usually only one cream shadow is used at a time, sometimes two. If you use more than two the eye looks muddy and the makeup is ineffective. Cream is also quick and effective for people who only have five minutes to do their makeup. Cream, when lavishly applied, can create a rich color statement to the eye for a dramatic look and is enhanced when powder shadow is blended into it. Cream eye shadows are often preferred by people with more mature eye skin or who desire a shadow that is easy to apply regardless of visual or physical limitations.
Frosty or Matte	Like lipsticks, shadows can be extremely matte with no shine because they do not enhance skin imperfections the way a frosty shadow can. The effect of matte shadows is like black and white photography. The look is akin to the powdery finish of photographs of movie stars between the 1920s and 1940s. Because matte shadows appear flat, they are the best formula of shadow to create very natural shading on the eye. They may also be completely frosty with undying shimmer and sparkle. These shadows electrify the eye and are usually a bolder type of color (bright blue, purple or burgundy, for example) These shadows can give almost a "wet" look to the eye and definitely captivate your makeup look. Many eye shadows have a subtle amount of shimmer in them that, when applied, acts as a light reflector and creates a smoother appearance to the eyes. This form of subtle shimmer or glow softly lights up the eye without stealing attention from the rest of the face. Often a single, subtle shimmer eye shadow all over the eye is all that is needed to create a fresh, soft and natural look. Matte or subtle shimmer is used more for a natural and finished look whereas a dramatic look can use any format of shadow.
Pencil	There are blunt tip, powder tip and felt-pen-like pencils that also serve as eye shadows. Some people have the most control with pencils, which makes penciled eye shadow very popular. Penciled shadows are a little more difficult to find, but several companies make them. These pencils come in all of the varying degrees of matte to frosty finishes previously mentioned.

Powder	Most eye shadows are powder so they can be easily and softly applied on the eye area and blend well with each other. It is important to feel the texture of the powder shadow with your finger. All makeup companies have varying amounts of pigment and creaminess to their powder shadows. It is in your best interest to find the highest pigment, most luxurious feeling shadows possible. You will know if they are high pigment because when you rub a small amount of shadow on your hand with your finger the color will actually intensify on your hand as you rub it. That means the color is rich in pigment and will achieve the longest lasting look throughout the day. You will know if a color is luxurious if it blends like a dream. Rub different colors of the eye shadow together on your hand. If they melt into each other beautifully, chances are they will blend as smoothly on your eye. Many of my clients complain that they are physically unable to make shadow blend. I suggest to them that perhaps the shadows they are using are physically unable to blend into each other. To make your life happier, find luxurious, high pigment shadows that do the work for you. Then all you need to do is wave your brush and the quality of the cosmetics will do their thing.
Gloss	A new trend for eyes is a glossy, wet look. Available in wands, pots or compacts, a small amount brushed over eye shadow or alone provides a trendy, hip finish. If used heavily, eye shadow will crease easily. As with any eye product, use only ophthalmologically tested products on your eyes. Lip gloss may give the same effect but can damage your eye. Definitely not worth it.

Cake	Cakes are pans of dry color that are water activated to achieve a liquid liner performance. Cake liners, though they require a little more preparation time, are generally more versatile and easier to use than liquid liners. You can achieve a highly refined or a dramatic line. The advantages are that they never dry out since their normal state is dry to begin with. They can also be softened or blended more easily to create different looks, and it is easier to clean up a mistake because the formula itself is not too intense. The only disadvantage of cake versus liquid is that you need water to activate the cake liner.
Liquid	Liquid liners come in a little bottle with a brush, in a mascara-type dispenser with a brush, or as a pen with the liquid flowing through a fine brush or ball point tip. You can achieve a highly refined or a dramatic line. Some liquid liners are waterproof and some are not. Most liquid liners require a little drying time before re-opening your eyes.
Pencil	Pencils are the most popular and most produced form of eyeliner. They can be cream based, which makes them ideal for creating a softer, smudged look to the eyeliner, and they can be waterproof to stand up to adverse weather or tears. Pencils produce softer, creamier looking lines for a more natural look, but can also be intensified and worn inside the lash line to create very dramatic (silent film like) makeup effects. Because pencils usually contain oil for softness to enhance ease of application, they are notorious for running and smudging throughout the day. You need to find a pencil that is neither too dry or too creamy if you want the effect of your pencil to endure throughout the day.
Shadow	Eye shadow can be used in place of any of these other forms of liners to line the eyes. Shadow liner usually has a softer look on the eye and can be used on top of another eyeliner to enhance its intensity and/or set the liner to prevent it from running. Some shadows can be activated with water to behave more like a cake liner. Generally speaking, shadow as liner creates less impact on the eye than all other forms of eye liners.

Mascara	Mascara thickens and generally intensifies the look of eyelashes. The most common colors of mascara are brown or black, and you can wear either depending on the look you want to achieve. Mascara also comes in almost any other color imaginable for more colorful and expressive makeup. Different mascaras boast particular features such as lengthening or thickening or conditioning. Decide for yourself what type of eyelashes your look requires and get the appropriate mascara. Most brands will offer you both waterproof and non-waterproof. If you don't need waterproof, it is best not to use it because you'll need special waterproof remover to get it off. Also, some waterproof mascaras are harsh on your lashes and can make them dry and brittle. (No fun!) Special tip: Navy mascara brightens the whites of your eyes. Really!

Mascara comes in these following forms.

Cream	The quickest, easiest, and most common form of mascara today comes pre-mixed in a tube with a wand. Be aware that once your wand touches your eye and goes back into the tube, bacteria from your eye has been introduced to the tube and will begin to breed immediately. Even though mascaras have anti-bacterial ingredients, the dark, moist environment inside the mascara tube is very fertile for bacteria. With that in mind, it is wise to get into the habit of changing your mascara tube every six weeks, whether it is running out or not. An infected eye is no fun and can be easily avoided.
Cake	The original mascara formula was cake. You added water to the dry pan of mascara color and mixed it up with your mascara brush until the formula became creamy. The advantage of this formula is that it never goes bad or dries out. The disadvantage is the fact that you have to mix it with water first. Cake mascara can make, by far, the thickest, most dramatic eyelash possible. In fact, If you wanted your lashes any thicker, you would have to use false eyelashes.

Now let's look at concealers, which are also referred to as cover-up.

Concealer

I consider concealer an eye makeup ingredient. However, if you are only wearing foundation without eye makeup, you would still want to use concealer to give the skin a finished appearance. Concealer either camouflages or neutralizes discoloration below the eye and anywhere else on the face.

The skin tissue around the eye is extremely thin and has only two layers of skin instead of three like the rest of the face. This thinness causes the eye area to become more transparent, thus exposing the blood and veins under the skin more easily. When eyes are strained or tired, pressure builds up and intensifies the natural darkness around the eye area. Concealer is like a third layer of skin that shields the inner darkness around the eye from showing through.

Let's first look at concealer as an eye makeup ingredient. After all your eye makeup is applied, a small amount of residual eye makeup usually falls below the eye. If you had already applied your concealer, you would remove it when cleaning up the residual eye makeup. If you have not already applied your concealer, you can simply remove the eye makeup residuals from below the eye, then apply the concealer for the first and only time.

If you do not wear eye makeup but want a generally even tone to your skin, then apply your concealer before applying your foundation for an even finish everywhere on the face.

Concealers come in wand, stick, or tube form and in light, medium, and dark shades. Make sure your concealer is the same intensity as your powder. Remember, concealers are all designed to do the same thing, so sample a few before buying.

Getting concealer to look natural on your face can be tricky. Often the concealer color doesn't match the face color or it emphasizes fine lines that otherwise would not be visible. I suggest blending a small amount of your foundation into your concealer before applying for two reasons: it makes the concealer match the rest of your face, and it creates a smoother finish under the eye. It also helps to moisturize the under-eye area well, which will provide a smoother base for the concealer.

There are color corrector concealers that come in the same shades as the color corrector powders listed in the foundation and powder section of this book. The same rules about corrective colors apply to concealers.

Eye Makeup Quick Look Guide

	Application	Advantages
EYEBROW		
Pencil	Draw On	Quick & Easy
Powder	Brush On	Fuller, Softer Look
EYE SHADOW BASE		
Cream	Brush or Finger	High Coverage
Powder	Brush or Puff	Soft Finish
EYE SHADOW		
Powder	Brush/Sponge Tip	Blend Many Colors
Cream	Finger, Brush	Quick, Long Lasting Color
Pencil	Draw On	Simplifies Application
Frost	All of the above	Glamorous, Flashy
Matte	All of the above	Softens Crepey Eyelids
EYELINER		
Pencil	Draw On	Quick, Smudgeable
Liquid	Brush On	High Definition Line
Cake	Brush On	Most Versatile
Eye shadow	Brush On	Softer Liner Look
MASCARA		
Cream	Brush On	Quick & Easy
Cake	Brush On	Thicker lashes, long lasting formula
CONCEALER		
Wand (cream)	Finger, Brush, Sponge	Quick & Easy
Stick (cream)	Finger, Brush, Sponge	Quick & Easy
Tube (cream)	Finger, Brush, Sponge	Quick & Easy
Pot (cream)	Finger, Brush, Sponge	Quick & Easy
Foundation	Finger, Brush, Sponge	Quick & Easy

A Touch of Cheek

I save cheeks for last. That way I don't apply too much color on the cheeks, compensating for lack of color before the lip and eye colors are applied. Cheek color, or blush, performs three important functions. First, cheek color frames the perimeter of your face and gives it a finished aura, much the same way a frame finishes a fine painting. Second, it enhances the natural shadow created by your cheek bone and creates the appearance of a perfectly lit facial structure. And third, it accentuates your facial contour, which gives your face more desired dimension

Your cheek color should be the same color base as your lip color (though not mandatory) and should be applied just under the peak of your natural cheek bone. Many women use their lipstick as their blush. There are also highlight cheek colors which lighten the upper part of the cheekbone, creating a higher looking cheekbone. Highlight cheek color should be blended above and below the contour cheek color. Also a soft, nearly translucent pink or peach blush applied to the apple of the cheek creates a healthy daytime glow on the face.

Blush is available in the following forms:

Cream	Cream blushes are usually blended on with your finger or a foundation sponge. They are good for dryer skins that tend to drink up cheek color. Cream blush can also be used as a base for powder blush to create a longer lasting cheek color or to create a dramatic effect. Cream blush comes in stick, pan or pencil form.
Powder	Powder blushes are the most popular form of cheek color. They are applied with a brush or cotton pad and smooth on easily for fast application.

Lipstick Quick Look Guide

Blush	Finish	Longetivity
Powder	Brush On	Blends Easily
Cream	Finger, Sponge	Long Lasting

Finishing with Technique

Once blush is applied, your application is complete. Now it's time to take a look at the whole picture and see what you have done. You should notice the whole person, not first this part, then that, etc. So when you assess your application, be objective and see if you have struck a balance between all your colors. One simple way to create balance is to make the center of your lower lip and the outer corner of your eye the same intensity. The colors don't need to be the same (and in most cases, won't be), but the intensity of the colors should be the same.

An excellent finishing technique is to mix a little concealer with a little foundation and "clean up" around your face. Clean-up can include correcting the lip line, trimming the eye brow and eyeliner, covering any blemish or other discoloration, etc. It is wise to make one more application of your translucent powder to veil and set the whole look. Avoiding eyes and lips, either brush on or press on one last layer of powder, then brush off any excess.

Maintaining Your Best Look Throughout the Day

Sure your makeup looks great, but how do you keep it looking great? If you applied your makeup adequately, you only need to carry a few items to maintain your look:

- lip color and liner

- compact powder with mirror

- powder puff and/or brush

- facial tissue

Some people feel better carrying every cosmetic they possibly can because maintaining a "fresh" look is important. I agree--nothing looks fresher than newly applied makeup. There are many excellent cosmetic bags. The list above should be enough to maintain your look without carrying an entire makeup counter with you wherever you go.

Tools of the Trade

The following items are tools you need in order to best apply your makeup.

Drug Store Products

Brush cleaner—a spray-on disinfectant cleaner for quick, daily maintenanc of your brushes

Cotton pads—to apply toner and powder and to remove eye makeup

Foundation sponge—to blend the foundation once it is applied by finger

Facial tissue—to clean and blot

Cotton swabs—to apply, clean and blend

Professional Products

Concealer brush—a synthetic bristle brush (natural fibers will absorb the oil in the concealer and become ruined) used to apply concealer and foundation to specific areas, ideal for finishing

Contour eye shadow brush—an angled or cone-shaped eye shadow brush for more specific shadow application, usually for darker colors in the crease of the eye

Eyebrow brush—to groom brows and to apply and blend brow color

Eyeliner brush—to apply liquid or cake liner, smudge pencil, and add shadow over eyeliner

Eye shadow brush—to generally apply eye shadow and blend different intensity shadows

Lip brush—to apply lip color and blend lip liner

Remember: "Good" makeup achieves a sense of balance on the face, meaning no particular feature stands out over the other

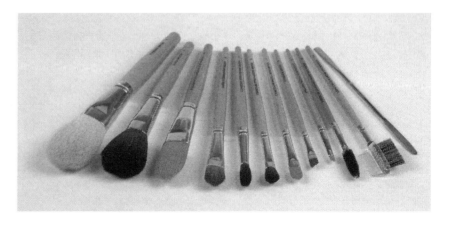

Blush brush—to apply blush as either contour, highlight or for a flushed look

Powder brush—to apply face powder and to remove excess powder

The first five items above can be found at any drug store. The other items, however, should be bought with care. Your brushes are an investment that will last far longer than any piece of makeup, and most quality brushes come with a lifetime guarantee. Your brushes are always on your face so choose the highest quality possible within your budget. The better tool can make a world of difference.

Trends and Other Passing Fancies

I regard trends as experiments that enable makeup to evolve. There will always be trends that reflect the emphasis of each particular fashion season. Trends are designed to be fun, extreme and temporary. Examples of makeup trends are matte lipstick, pearlescent foundation, all frost colors or all matte colors, provocative color combinations, full brows, no brows, full lips, no lips, dark eyes, no eyes, etc. Trends are endless. They wake up your makeup and keep fashion fresh.

I suggest that you first get the makeup items that support a majority of your cosmetic needs. Once that is accomplished, you can feel free to experiment with a trendy lip or eye color or whatever is hot for the season. It is safe to say that not every trend is appropriate for every individual and being fashionable and looking your best do not always go hand in hand.

Trends go out as fast as they come in, so don't let them overwhelm your good sense. A trend that involves shaving off your eyebrows, for example, will be temporary, but the loss of your eyebrows won't!

Remember: Trends go out as fast as they come in, so don't let them overwhelm your good sense.

Answers to Frequently Asked Questions

What are all those ingredients in my cosmetics?

It truly takes a chemist to recognize and understand all the ingredients listed on a box of moisturizer or eye shadow. If it is necessary for the consumer to have this in-depth knowledge, there are a couple of good publications that can tell you exactly what each ingredient is, its derivative, and possible side effects. For people with low allergic tolerance to products, this method of ingredient shopping can save you time, money and a terrible skin reaction.

If products tend to bother your skin, yet you want to use them anyway, I suggest visiting a dermatologist who is cosmetic savvy. It is vital for you to find out what it is exactly that your skin is allergic to, then avoid any products that contain those ingredients.

As far as products being dermatologically tested, there isn't a product in the department store that hasn't been tested. It is standard operational procedure to skin test any cosmetic before investing in it and putting it on the market. There are some lines that announce that their products are dermatologically tested to highlight that point (Clinique, for instance). It is smart marketing on Clinique's part to point out how concerned they are about the healthfulness of their product. It attracts many consumers with problem skin who can't afford to take chances. That is their selling point. That is why their salespeople wear lab coats as uniforms, to look informed and tested. However, all products have undergone virtually the same testing. There are still people who have reactions when they use Clinique products. It is not because Clinique is a bad brand of cosmetics; it is because everyone is allergic to something. It doesn't matter what dermatologically tested brand of cosmetics you use, if you are allergic or sensitive to a particular ingredient, you will have a reaction. That is why I stress figuring out with a dermatologist what it is you are allergic to before buying more cosmetics.

How do I know which products are safe for me to use?

1. Sample everything before you buy it. Apply samples like foundation or moisturizer near the jaw line so if you do have a reaction it is not in a noticeable part of the face. Use small amounts of color (lipstick, eye shadow, blush, etc.) at first to see if there is a reaction. If there is no reaction, slowly increase the amount you use until you have reached your desired cosmetic effect.

2. When purchasing, though you may want everything, start very small. For instance, instead of buying into a sophisticated and complicated skincare system, buy just the facial moisturizer. Use it for a week and pay attention to the results. If you like what you see and there are no side effects, go back and try the eye cream. It is far safer to slowly build on the line. This way if you begin to have any kind of a negative reaction, it is easier to single out the product that is causing the irritation.

If you start using five new products on your skin and you have a reaction, it is far more difficult to discern where the problem lies. When this happens, the consumer usually returns everything and has to start all over again. Four out of the five products might have been really good for her but since she doesn't know which product was the bad apple, they all become "bad" products and the consumer thinks there is nothing out there she can use that won't cause a reaction. Out of frustration, this consumer will buy five new products from a different line and end up having some kind of a reaction.

This can become a nightmare cycle for the consumer and can be easily avoided. Start small and slowly build on a line. If you have a reaction to a product, find out through your dermatologist which ingredient in particular caused the allergic reaction. Then avoid products that contain that ingredient.

A repeat offender ingredient that is often the cause of skin irritation is mineral oil. Mineral oil is the best known ingredient to give a product "slip" (the ease with which it goes on to the skin). The problem is that there are so many products that use mineral oil. What's a girl to do? Except for the most extremely sensitive skin (a very small minority), there is mineral oil that your skin can tolerate. It all comes back to the quality of ingredients.

When you have your oil changed in your car, you have your choice of what weight of oil to use. Cosmetic manufacturers have that same choice with mineral oil. Some will use the least expensive, heavier weight mineral oil (such as Revlon or Cover Girl). The problem is, if you are sensitive to mineral oil, the heavier the weight the more sensitive you will be. Then there are more expensive and refined lines (Yves St. Laurent, Chanel, Christian Dior) that also use mineral oil; however, the oil they use is highly refined and of the highest grade so that skin that is sensitive to mineral oil can use these products without side effects.

Alcohol is similar to mineral oil in the sensitivity classification. The grade of alcohol determines whether the sensitive individual will have a reaction. In cleansing products, alcohol kills bacteria that can cause skin to break out. In cosmetics, alcohol helps products set quickly to the skin. In a crude analogy, it is like drinking alcohol. Cheaper forms of alcohol (malt liquor, Thunder Bird) can cause severe headaches. More refined alcohols (like Courvoisier or Johnny Walker) can be kinder the morning after because they are a more refined, higher quality product that the body can more easily assimilate. That is not to say that if you drink malt liquor you will get a headache or if you drink Courvoisier you won't. Everyone has a different tolerance level. On the whole, however, the higher the quality of alcohol, the kinder it treats your system, and the same goes with alcohol on your face. Harsh, strong alcohol will burn, dry and damage the skin. Refined alcohol will cleanse, clear and protect the skin.

Can I detect potentially harmful ingredients from the product's packaging?

Most definitely! For instance, too much oil in any product can give even the sturdiest of skins problems after repeated use. Check to see what the first few ingredients are in every product. Remember that ingredients are listed in order of amount, the first ingredient being the highest percentage ingredient present in the product. If the product lists any kind of oil, lanolin, or alcohol as it's first four ingredients, even though the presence of these ingredients are part of good cosmetics, it indicates that the product may cause irritation due to the high percentage of these ingredients. A little of each is good, but a lot of each is too much and will probably cause you problems. Also, the absence of ingredients indicates that this product is simplified and maybe not highly effective. Unfortunately, it usually takes a chemistry degree to fully understand the ingredient listing on most cosmetics. Here are three comprehensive guides to cosmetic ingredients:

A Consumer's Dictionary of Cosmetic Ingredients by Ruth Winter

Milady's Skincare and Cosmetic Ingredients Dictionary by Natalia Michalun, M. Varinia Michalun

What's in Your Cosmetics? A Complete Consumer's Guide to Natural and Synthetic Ingredients by Aubrey Hampton

What's the truth about animal testing?

It is an area of concern for many consumers that the brand of cosmetics they use does not test on animals. There are some lines that even advertise that they are animal-test-free products. All of this is admirable but there is a truth behind all cosmetics. Until recently, if it went on your face, it was tested on an animal according to FDA rules. However, it is no longer the case that cosmetics, by law, need to be animal tested. Most cosmetic companies have adopted a cruelty-free policy. Be aware that even though certain products claim to be cruelty free, the company may still practice animal testing on other products. For up-to-date information on who tests and who doesn't, contact:

People for the Ethical Treatment of Animals
501 Front Street
Norfolk, VA 23501
757-622-PETA (7382)

What can you learn about a product by reading its claims?

Because cosmetics are only legally allowed to act upon the epidermis (the outermost layer of skin), whatever claims it makes are temporary ones. Since skin replenishes itself continuously on a 21-28 day cycle, whatever temporary results you have achieved using a particular product must be maintained with that product to maintain the results. There are no long lasting cures sold at the cosmetic counter. There are excellent short term benefits.

As skincare technology increases, consumers are seeing greater results in a shorter amount of time. There are no miracles out there, yet there are some fine products that can produce positive results in a short amount of time. A word of caution: don't immediately use the strongest formula of whatever you are using (alpha-hydroxy, retin-A, etc.) More is definitely not better and in many cases can do more harm than good. Be sensible when you find an ingredient that produces great results for your skin. Slowly upgrade to stronger strengths if you want greater results. Too much of a good thing can turn into a bad thing real quick on your skin.

Which cosmetic companies have the most/fewest complaints?

This may seem a little too obvious but the bigger the company, the more the complaints. This is directly caused by numbers. The more people use a product, the more problems arise. The ratio of total consumers to total complaints is constant. Remember that we are concerning ourselves with department store quality products only. Using drug store cosmetics regularly is equivalent to eating fast food every day. The first couple of days it feels the same as higher quality food. Then it starts to take its toll on your body.

Department stores protect their interest by carrying cosmetics that are not available anywhere else at a discounted price. All department store cosmetics are regulated and are the same price no matter where you buy them. Consequently, the cosmetics found in department stores have passed a certain quality standard to be offered at the department store level. The department store has weeded out the potential "lemon" lines that will give you problems at every turn. Once at the department store it is up to you, the consumer, to use your good judgment and common sense when buying cosmetics. That is why the information in this book does not tell you what to buy, rather, how to buy.

Can I trust small or upstart companies?

Yes you can, as long as the department store endorses their quality and offers a money back guarantee on whatever you buy. The science of making good cosmetics is common knowledge among cosmetic manufacturers. Manufacturers know what ingredients make the best quality cosmetics. They also know where and where not to make less expensive ingredient substitutions without compromising the end result too dramatically. As with any cosmetic purchase, what should guide your buying instinct is if the product in question appears to fulfill your needs. If it does, get it.

The hard part is resisting temptation. You may find salespeople you really like helping you with your purchase. They make further recommendations. Based on their appeal you buy more products. You then spend three times as much as you thought you would on products that sounded good at the time of purchase.

How does price figure into a product's worth?

Again, let it be known that the standard mark-up for cosmetics is 500%. Once that is accepted, there is a difference in quality compared to price up to a point. I firmly believe that the more expensive (designer) products are the better products. Will another brand do? Of course it will. It is up to you to decide for yourself what things you want the best in. For some it is cars, for others clothes or wine or perfume or whatever. And there are those who only want the best cosmetics. Dollar for dollar, the designer makeup isn't that much better than other makeup. Half the extra amount you pay for designer cosmetics is for the quality, and the other half is the name. You cannot get one without the other.

The products that are the most important in terms of quality are:

· moisturizer

· foundation

· powder

Everything else is a matter of taste.

What are my favorites?

Despite my attempts at instructing you how to buy the best products for you, there are still those who don't have the time or interest to invest in their cosmetic shopping. For these individuals, and as well as for general knowledge, I will list some of the most popular and proven lines and products.

Every year and intermittently Allure and Marie Claire magazines run the top cosmetic products of the year (other magazines have similar lists, but I find these two the most reputable). These are excellent guides to what has been tried and proven effective on the cosmetic-using public. I read these lists every year to keep current with new products as they develop. These lists are a must read.

All right, my favorites! I will list in order of usage.

Skincare: Borghese, Chanel, Clarins, Shiseido

Foundation & Powder: Chanel, Ge, Yves Saint Laurent

Lipstick & Blush: Every type except for super matte, all-day lipstick. They do way more damage than good.

Eye Makeup : Chanel, Christian Dior, Nars, MAC, Yves Saint Laurent

Brushes: Lorac, Mac, Make-up Gourmet, Shu Uemura, Trish McEvoy

How can consumers avoid buying all new makeup with each season's new trends?

Each season's trend is usually an accent on a particular part of the face, such as dewy skin, red lips, thicker brows, etc. If you wish to stay in style, my suggestion is to pick out a trend product or two that creates the season's look, such as pearl foundation base, red lipstick, eyebrow pencil or powder, and buy it from an economical line such as MAC or Clinique.

If you end up loving the look and want to incorporate it into an everyday look, then buy the similar product from your line of preference. If you end up tiring of the trend and find the look has no lasting appeal for you, you have spent a minimal amount to be in style and to discover a part of your makeup that doesn't work for you.

How do I know which trends to follow?

You don't. Treat trends as ideas. That's why I suggest experimenting cheaply before investing in a completely new look. The advantage of trends is that you will discover little tricks that make you feel more attractive (many of my clients are elated to discover what an eyebrow pencil can do for them).

In time, as trends repeat themselves in different forms, you will have prior knowledge upon which to base your experimentation.

I once trained in the martial arts. My instructor, after teaching me all the correct kicks, blocks, punches, maneuvers and in what order to deliver them, said to me "Forget everything and do what comes natural." The lesson I learned is that the end result of any system is that there is no system. You can only fill your head with so much knowledge, then it is up to you, the individual, to allow your instincts to act upon that knowledge.

Please forgive my "snatch the pebble from my hand" metaphor. I want to free you from the idea of the "right and wrong" approach to make up. Makeup should always be based on personal choice. As Janis Joplin clearly stated "You know you got it (scream) if it makes you feel good!"

Remember: These are lines that I particularly like and that work for me. Everyone has specific tastes and will favor one products over another.

Conclusion

I hope that this reading has been valuable to you. The information I have shared with you is designed to help you find the best skincare products for you and to coordinate your cosmetic purchases to create the makeup looks you desire. The next step, of course, is to *apply* your new cosmetics. It's smart to have your makeup done many times in department stores by different people to learn new techniques.

There are also many books that will help answer many of your makeup application questions. I will be writing a book of my personal makeup application techniques, and if you found this book helpful, I am sure you will enjoy my next one as much, if not more.

I also want to say that makeup is a very individual expression. There are no wrongs in applying makeup. I find makeup to be very honest. We put it right on our face where everyone can see it. To this purpose, makeup can become an extension of our lifestyle and personality. The beauty of makeup is that it washes off. The next time you are feeling extraordinary, try a new makeup look to match. Thank you for reading and have fun shopping.

Contact Information

To order more copies of the *Cosmetic Counter Survival Guide*, or to contact me personally with questions or comments, please visit me online at *chris@makeupgourmet.com* or *www.makeupgourmet.com*.